The Magic of Yogurt

For Cooking and Beauty

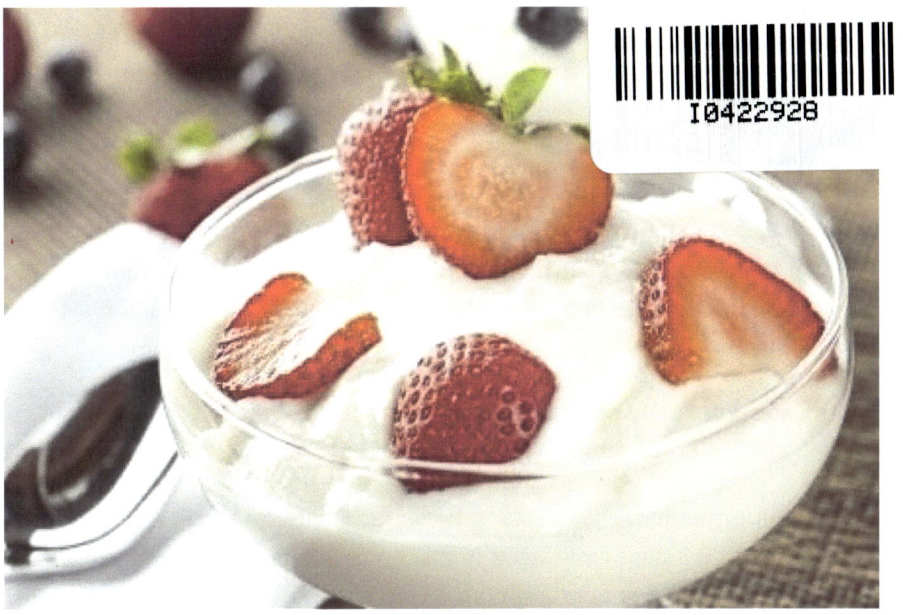

Dueep Jyot Singh

Natural Remedy Series

Mendon Cottage Books

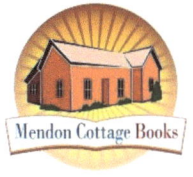

JD-Biz Publishing

Our books are available at

1. Amazon.com
2. Barnes and Noble
3. Itunes
4. Kobo
5. Smashwords
6. Google Play Books

Table of Contents

Introduction

Nobody really knows who first discovered yogurt. Butter is supposed to have been discovered millenniums ago, when camel's milk was placed in animal skin hides while being transported from one place to another by Arab or Turkish nomads. The ambulatory movement of the camel walking across the desert seem to have a churning effect on the hides, and in the evening, when the milk was taken out of the sack, two new products were discovered. Butter and buttermilk.

This possibly apocryphal serendipity is on par with the supposed discovery of wine. Millenniums ago, a Greek slave was suffering from toothache, and that was so painful that she found an earthenware pitcher full of fermenting grape juice left by some other careless slave. All those bubbles made her think that it was poison, and she would rather drink that, than suffer the pain of a toothache. So she did drink of the juice of the grape and fell asleep. And the miracle of wine was discovered to gladden the hearts of generations. No wonder the Greeks had a God Bacchus – also known as Dionysus and the Roman equivalent Liber to whom you liberally paid libations, before you drank wine – for wine.

But nobody has told us how yogurt was discovered and by whom. But in ancient Indian medicine texts, the mixture of honey with yogurt eaten every day is considered to be the food of the gods to keep you everlastingly healthy.

Along with yogurt, the side products of bacterially fermented milk included buttermilk and butter. Every house proud woman made sure that she kept some yogurt back from yesterday's batch to prepare today's batch of yogurt.

These cultures have enzymes and bacteria, which are extremely beneficial for your digestive system.

The enzymes produce lactic acid. Lactic acid is what is going to ferment the lukewarm milk. It is also what makes your yogurt sour if you leave it in a warm place after the yogurt has been made. So the moment you see the yogurt set, put it in a cool place.

The milk which are normally used to make yogurts all over the world down the ages have included, Dri milk [a yak is male. The female is called a Dri.], goats milk, cow's milk, camels milk, mare milk and milk from buffaloes and ewes. Of this, cow's milk is most easily available, even though there are companies who are producing yogurt made from soya milk.

The generic name Yogurt is derived from the Turkish word yugurmak – to Curdle-you may also call it yaghourt or jogourt if you are in Europe. The term yogourt is used to order yogurt in French.

In Persian mythology, Abraham said that it was a regular intake of yogurt, which kept him healthy, and promoted longevity as well as fecundity. This idea is still prevalent in the East, and that is why yogurt is a part of every luncheon or breakfast cuisine, as far as possible, in the Orient. Maybe that is why the population growth in these areas was so much, in ancient times.

In fact, I remember one of my friends' mother feeding us kids ready on the way to the examination hall with a bowl full of yogurt and honey. According to her, that would keep our mind cool, and we would not be confused. We eager and perpetually hungry team, made sure that her house was the last stop – while picking up the five members of the gang on way to school, – because we would be blessed and fed yogurt and honey by her mom. How come our moms never did that? But we never told them that.

According to the French, Francis the first suffered a lot from stomach problems, including diarrhea. His French medical men were at their wits sends until this news was conveyed to one of his allies the Persian King, Suleiman The Magnificent. He immediately sent his hakim, which cured the king with yogurt. And the yogurt became an integral part of French cuisine.

A company in Prague was the first one to add some fruit jam to yogurt, and patented this recipe in 1933. That is why; most of the yogurts you find in the market today have some pieces of fruit added to them. But this traditional idea of adding something to the yogurt was in vogue in Eastern cuisine for millenniums in the form of Raita and cucumber dips.

It has been found that many people who are lactose intolerant, have managed to digest yogurt without any side effects. This is due to the bacteria and the lactic acid.

Yogurts are rich in vitamins B6 and B12, proteins, riboflavin, and calcium.

Shopping for Yogurt

I was walking down a shopping aisle, in a supermarket, and I was amazed to see so many different brands of yogurt, some with fruits added, some with artificial flavorings, some yogurt brands calling themselves Swiss yogurt, and with lots of impressing information about their probiotic bacteria content.

Okay, I am going to rain on your parade, now. All those artificially packed yogurt containers may have artificial preservatives, and flavorings, and other such items in them, which you may think are healthy. But they are definitely not so.

Real yogurt is the one which you make at home. But most of us are so busy, that we absolutely forget to take five minutes out every evening before we switch off the light in the kitchen, and thus we reach for the nearest flavored yogurts. In fact, most of us lunch off yogurts in banana and strawberry flavor.

Well, you are eating something, which you find tasty. But is that real yogurt, made from cow's milk or is it a mixture of soybean milk with the preservation to lengthen its shelf life?

Should You Invest in a Yogurt Maker?

My Yanqui cousin says that it is necessary in her kitchen, because she is an extremely busy, busy, busy person. But then, she also loves the latest techno gadgets! Some yogurt makers come with different flavors. So one day she has strawberry, the other day she has banana. But she makes the yogurt herself.

These yogurt makers have temperature control. They also make yogurt really quickly. Cuisinart gives you good yogurt makers, but all the yogurt makers out there are highly priced. Besides this, remember that people have been making yogurt for centuries without technical gadgets.

Look for deals on eBay; you can get them from prices ranging from USD27 to above. Buy a really huge and expensive one if you make enough of yogurt every day to feed a hotel. For a small family, do it the traditional way! Gardeners yogurt maker is for USD29.95.

How to Make the Perfect Yogurt

You make yogurt in the East in this traditional way. Normally, milk is boiled in India, even though you get it pasteurized. Because traditionally, Indians do not trust the pasteurizing process and would rather boil it again before use, than drink it straight from the milk bottle or from the packet.

So boil 1 L of milk. Allow to cool until it is lukewarm. You are going to see a thin layer of cream floating on top. You can keep it to add some taste you are making yogurt.

You need 3 tablespoons full of yogurt culture. What is yogurt culture? It is just the remainder of the yogurt, which was left behind after you finished the yogurt you made yesterday. Remember to keep at least 2 to 3 tablespoons full and do not empty out that yogurt bowl.

Dip your finger in the milk. If it is tolerably warm, in the warm weather, this is the time you put in the yogurt. Whip it briskly with a spoon, cover with a lid, and placed by one side of the stove in your warm kitchen. This is normally made overnight, so that you have perfect yogurt to eat for breakfast the next morning. The next morning, it has set, so put it in the fridge.

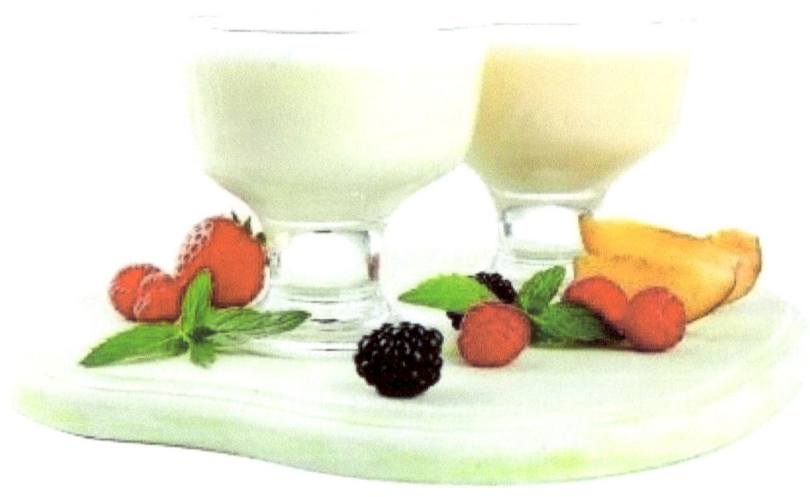

If you really want a traditional taste, boil this milk in a red earthenware pot, allow it to cool to lukewarm, add the culture, and leave the yogurt to set. This is considered to be one of the most delicious ways in which to eat milk products and meat products in India, and also in other countries in the East –

cooking in earthenware pots. This yogurt is going to have the taste of mother Earth, in a sweetened form. I still cannot understand how that yogurt got sweet. I never added any sugar to it. It is also going to have a distinctly delicious wet earthenware aroma.

Also, I found a friend setting yogurt in cold weather, – freezing Missouri weather – by warming up her oven at 125°C for five minutes. Then she put in the yogurt container in the oven and left it overnight. Good idea!

How to Prevent the Yogurt from Getting Watery

Have you just spooned off a chunk of yogurt, only to find the rest of it turning watery? This is going to happen when you cut into the yogurt, just like you were cutting into a pie or into the cake. The best way to prevent your beautifully set yogurt from getting watery is to spoon off the yogurt, layer by layer. That means that you are spooning off the set yogurt instead of breaking it. That breaking process means you are mixing it with its watery composition and component.

Yogurt in Cuisine

Yogurt is the best diet food for babies, as well as for old people because it is so easily digested and keeps your system healthy. If you are suffering from: problems, try eating lots of yogurt. This is going to cure your tummy ailments.

Yogurt – Cucumber soup – Tarator

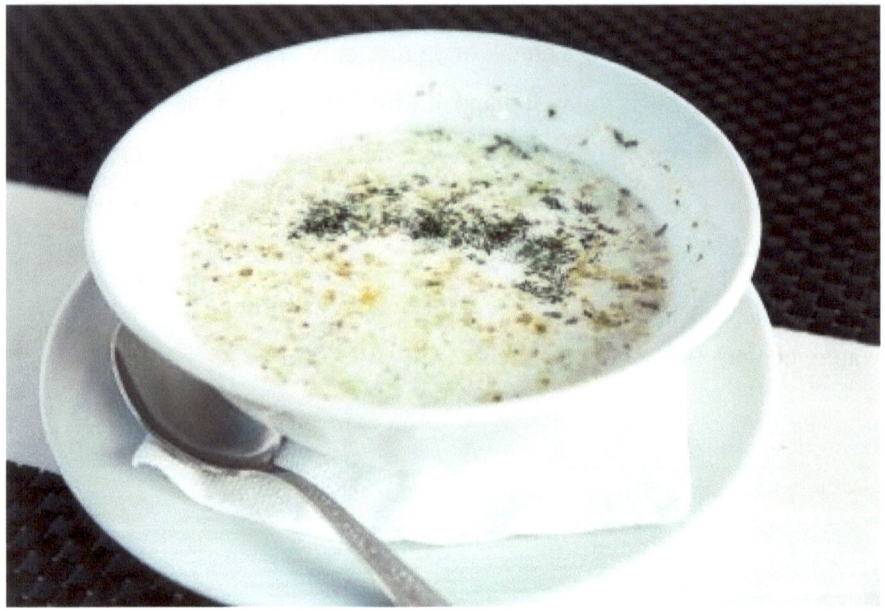

This is a traditional Belgian soup/salad dip.

For this you need 500 g of yogurt, two cucumbers grated, some dill, salt, pepper, garlic, salad oil and walnuts.

Mix the cucumber with the yogurt, add some water, and mix really well. Chop the dill, and added to this yogurt cucumber mixture. Crush the garlic and add it. Do the same to the walnuts and sprinkle it on top of the mixture. Add salt and salad oil, and your Tarator is ready for serving.

Funnily enough, the same thing is called Tarator in Lebanon, and it is also made in the same way and used as a dip. East and West, but the dish remains the same.

When you add a couple of boiled egg yolks to it, as garnish, it turns into a Russian yogurt soup called Okroshka!

Raita

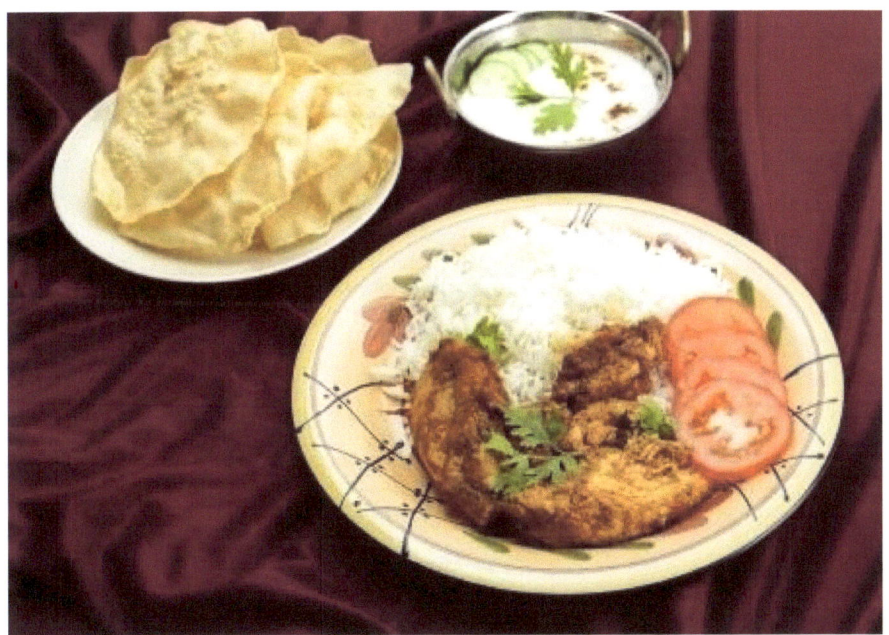

Raita is necessary, especially when you are eating highly spiced meat!

This is the traditional accompaniment to dishes, along with salads. Ordinary yogurt on its own is called da-hi (pronounced duh-heen) in the Indian subcontinent.

1 cup of yogurt.

Two medium sized tomatoes, chopped up.

One onion, chopped up.

Half a cucumber chopped up.

Mint to decorate.

Rocksalt, pepper, roasted cumin seeds and chili powder for taste.

Sprinkle the salt on the cut cucumber. Chop up the onions and tomatoes together and shred the mint.

Squeeze out the juice of the cucumber. Whisk the yogurt with a fork or in your blender, and add all the chopped vegetables with the spices.

Sprinkle the shredded mint over this yogurt and mix well. You can serve this cooled or at room temperature.

I have to make this for lunch every day in the summers. The onion protects me from sunstroke. The cucumber cools my system and keeps me well hydrated.

You may also want to try other raita combinations with onions and chopped boiled potatoes. This cooling lunch accompaniment is also delicious as a snack on its own when you are not feeling like a heavy lunch in the summer.

Try this as a dip for pieces of vegetables.

Mishti doi (literally sweet yogurt)

Just add 2 tablespoons of honey to the yogurt milk, when you are making the yogurt to have instant sweet yogurt. Mishit doi is something else, and was one thing which I loved eating when I visited the eastern parts of the Indian subcontinent.

Every Bengali or Eastern housewife here, feeds her family with Mishti doi – with lots of cream – regularly.

The traditional dish is made by boiling 1 L of creamy milk over low heat until it has been reduced to half of its volume. Do not allow the milk to scorch. Allow it to cool, until it is lukewarm.

Now take 250 g of sugar, add four tablespoons full of honey, and heat on low heat, until the sugar has been caramelized. Now add this sugar to the milk. Add 4 tablespoons full of yogurt culture. Put this in an earthenware pot, and allow setting in a warm place.

Serve chilled.

Yogurt as Tenderizer

Yogurt can also be used as a marinade and a meat tenderizer for tough meat. Instead of using papain, just put the meat in yogurt, with some cloves of crushed garlic, salt, pepper, red chilies and placed in the refrigerator for 24 hours. You have delicious, tender meat now.

Chicken in Yogurt

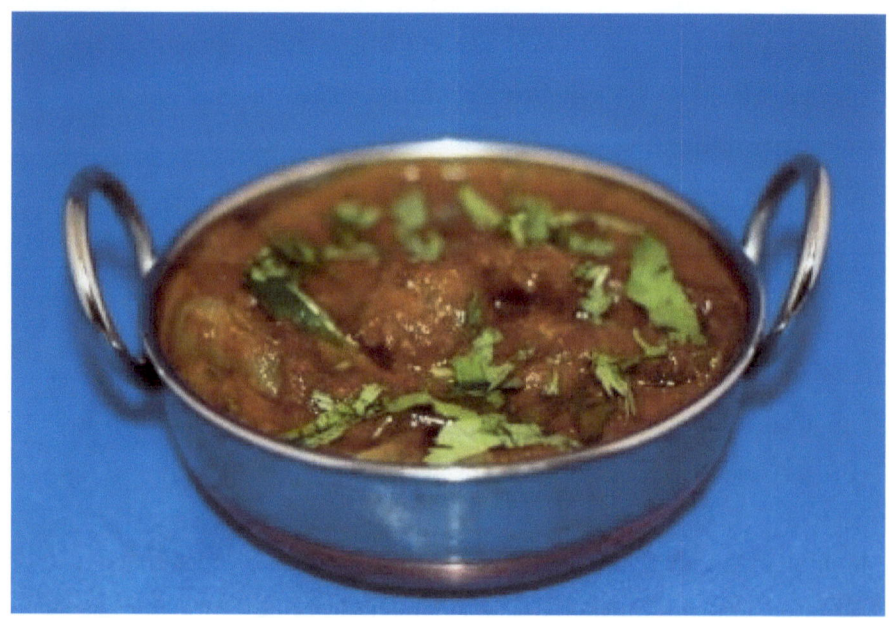

You are going to get a rich, creamy gravy, thanks to the yogurt.

Ingredients :

2 ½ pounds chicken, cut into bite sized pieces.

2 ½ tablespoons full clarified butter-desi ghee.

12 ounces yogurt

One large pimento

2 inches green ginger, grated

Three green chilies crushed.

16 large cloves of garlic, crushed

5 tablespoons full, minced coriander, cilantro or parsley leaves

1 teaspoon paprika and salt to taste.

Wash the jointed chicken. Prick all over with a very sharp fork. Beat the yogurt with the pimento, greens, ginger, paprika, chilies, garlic, and salt, and make a marinade. The garlic is not too much; the yogurt counteracts its pungency and power.

Marinate the chicken in this yogurt marinade for 12 hours in the refrigerator.

Heat a Wok until it is hot. Now throw in the chicken and marinade so that it makes a steam – making splash when it touches the bottom of the pan. Stir in the parsley. Cover immediately. Cook on high heat for four – five minutes, then on medium heat until the yogurt is dry, except for a little gravy at the bottom. Do not let this get brown.

Stir the chicken to coat it evenly. If you want the chicken to be light-colored, serve hot at this point with rice. If you want it to be deeper Brown, draw the pan half of the heat, and ladle all the sauce onto the chicken. All the contents are pushed to one side of the pan. In the middle of the pan, melt the clarified butter and roll the chicken in it gently, without browning. Serve hot with all the tasty scrapings from the sides of the Wok.

Just love "them" scrapings. What a pity cooks throw them away in hotels, because they do not add to the final good looks and presentation of a delicious chicken in yogurt.

Making Whey at Home

What is whey? That is the product left over, when you remove all the liquid content from yogurt. You can either solidify it and eat it chopped up and fried, or you can use it as a spicy dip.

Take 3 pints of homemade yogurt unsweetened.

Keep the yogurt in a warm place for about two days. Normally I recommend putting it in a cool place so that it does not go sour. But we want something really fermented and tasty.

Now add half a cup of water to this yogurt, and blend it in your blender along with the salt. You may find the water separating from the solid yogurt. Continue blending till you have a blended liquid. Now place this in a pan, and boil on low heat so that the milk solid becomes a solid lumpy mass.

Traditionally, the yogurt is drained on layers of cheese cloth. So place the yogurt in cheesecloth, and make a knot at the ends. My grandmother used to sling this yogurt over a tap, and place a utensil underneath. Then she used to leave it overnight. By morning, all the liquid would have collected in the utensil. If you do not have a cheesecloth around, you can also try draining with a drainer with a very fine mesh. If you are draining through a mesh, place some weight over the yogurt.

Let the dried whey dry a little more, before you solidify it in cubes in the fridge. Pack them up in watertight bags.

Do not throw away that water. That is delicious, when you added to gravies, to thicken the masala or the soup. It is going to give the food a sour tangy taste.

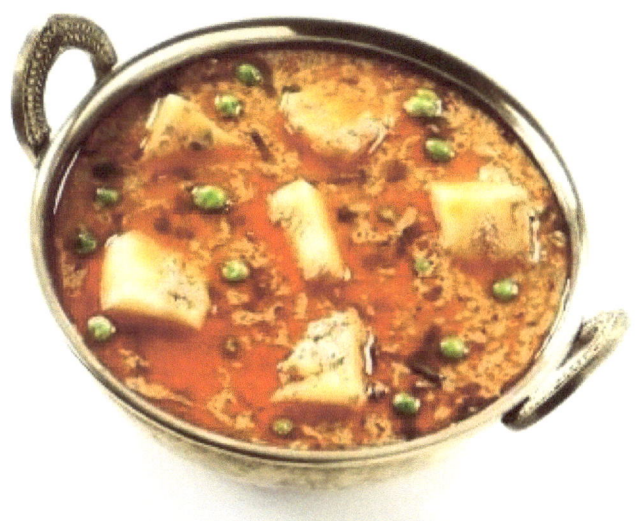

Stirfried pieces of fried whey with potatoes and peas in a rich gravy. This is the staple dish in many north Indian households called aloo mattar paneer tarri- literally potato, Peas, cheesecake curry.

Buttermilk or Lassi

This is the traditional refreshing drink in many parts of the East, and though we do not use this in cookies, as is done in many parts of the West, including the USA, buttermilk is drunk in large quantities as a standalone refreshing drink in the summer.

How Do You Make Traditional Buttermilk

2 cups rich creamy yogurt.

2 Equal amount of crushed ice or iced water.

Two table spoons honey

Pepper and salt to taste

Half a teaspoonful of roasted roughly ground cumin seeds

Since ancient times in the East, when there were no mixers and blenders around, all these items were placed in a huge churn and churned by hand until the mixture was frothy. The side product was of course fresh butter, which would then be scooped off and placed in clay containers.

This buttermilk was then topped off with a slice of cream or yogurt and served as an excellent digestive, with lunch in summer, or just drunk whenever you feel thirsty, to prevent you from getting dehydrated in the hot summer sun.

If you are in the South of India, and want buttermilk, you are going to get **Moru** in the summer. It is just plain buttermilk, with salt, spices, Curry leaves and mustard added to keep you well refreshed and dehydrated.

Yogurt for Beauty

Curing Dandruff

Also, they told me that my dandruff condition, if I had any, would disappear if I made a mixture of yogurt and lemon juice, and rubbed it in my scalp, before shampooing. Believe me, it works. So throw away your chemical-based shampoo, and try this natural remedy to get rid of dandruff.

Yogurt as a Hair Conditioner

When I used to travel in the North of India, I noticed that the ladies had long silky lustrous hair, but they also had a characteristic ferment-y smell around them. I soon found out the reason.

They were using yogurt as a hair conditioner before shampooing. They used to mix yogurt with mustard oil, and then ask one of their relatives to do a scalp massage with this odoriferous mixture while they roasted in the sun. The smell is enough to put any sensitive nose off and one would not want to be in the vicinity of cooking mustard oil and curds in the summer sun. Yes, I went through it, and let me tell you, that my hair remained manageable for two weeks after this massage and conditioning.

Yogurt as a Facemask

Also, I wondered what kept their skin so soft, fair and smooth. The answer was a regular facemask of honey, yogurt, and turmeric, and oatmeal applied instead of soap to their skin to keep it white, well moisturized, soft and appealing. But what about the smell. Quoth I. Would I not stink of stale yogurt? Not if I had a shower after 20 minutes, after I had exfoliated my skin of all its dirt. After the bath they moisturized their skins with almond oil or rosewater.

Rosewater for Beauty

All right, I am repeating the recipe for rosewater, even though I have put it in many other of my beauty remedy books. That is because it is much better making rosewater at home than to buy it from shops. The product you buy in the shop is going to be distilled water with some drops of rose oil extract, giving you a beautiful rosewater perfume. It is better you make rosewater right at home.

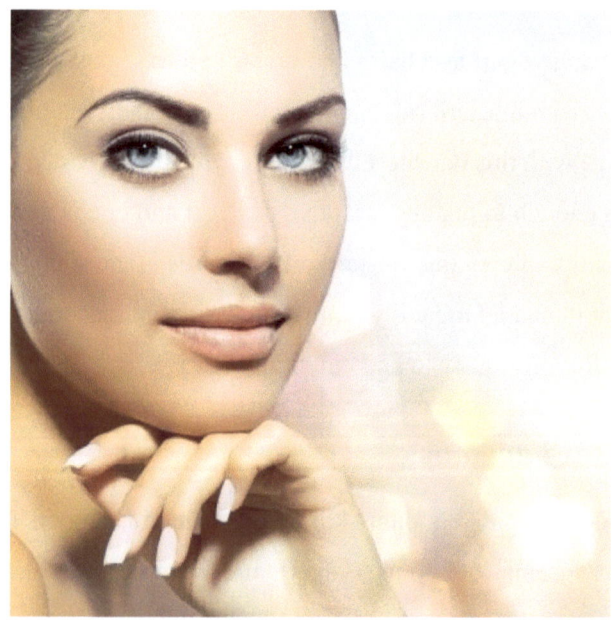

Rosewater honey and yogurt facemasks are going to keep your skin smooth and lovely.

I normally use this as a liquid base, when I want to make facemasks.

How To Make Rose Water

Rosewater is normally available in markets at exorbitant prices, but in India, anybody with access to the red rose - Rosa Damascena and a little bit of time enjoys making Rosewater at home. This Rosewater is used in cosmetics, as well as in cookery to impart the flavor of the Rose to your meal or to your skin.

Ingredients needed- 1 Cup Rose petals - 12 to 14 flowers.
2 cups water
Lots of ice.
A huge cooking pan - pan number one - with lid in which another pan - pan number two - can be placed comfortably.

Rosewater is just a matter of distillation. Put a wire stand in pan number one, on which you are going to stand the other pan number two. The condensed Rosewater is going to fall into pan number two.

Place the petals at the bottom of the pan number one. Now, cover the petals with water. Place pan number two on the wire stand. Now take the lid and place it upside down on pan number one, thus effectively covering the Rose petals, pan number two and the water. The Rose water is going to condense when you place the blocks and chunks of ice on the inverted lid.

You are going to have a cupful of precious distilled Rosewater, after 25 minutes of slow steaming of the Rose petals.

Precautions - Remember to have enough of water to cover the Rose petals. Also, it should not be of such a large quantity, that it displaces the wire stand.

This cooled water is now pure Rosewater. Pour it in a sterilized glass bottle. Use it to your heart's content. You may see a little bit of oil swimming over the surface of the water. This is Rose oil, and is even more precious. So if you used lots of petals in a larger pan, you may find even more Rose oil.

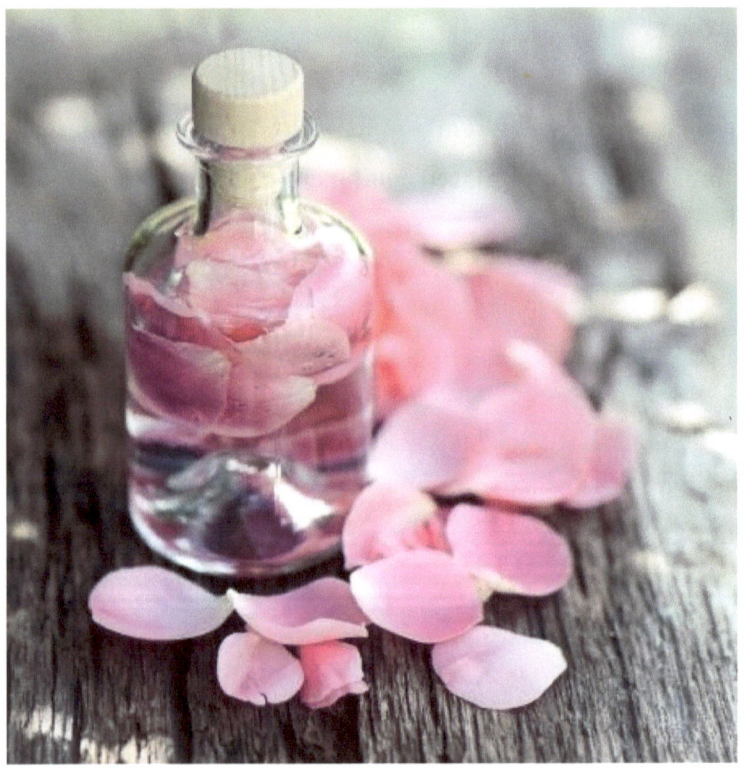

Conclusion

I have not touched the healing recipes of yogurt, because I am not sure whether they work especially as personal douches and getting rid of fungal infections. That is why, the magic of yogurt is concentrating only on yogurt-based dishes, and how you can keep beautiful with it.

Author Bio

Dueep Jyot Singh is a Management and IT Professional who managed to gather Postgraduate qualifications in Management and English and Degrees in Science, French and Education while pursuing different enjoyable career options like being an hospital administrator, IT,SEO and HRD Database Manager/ trainer, movie scriptwriter, theatre artiste and public speaker, lecturer in French, Marketing and Advertising, ex-Editor of Hearts On Fire (now known as Solsctice) Books Missouri USA, advice columnist and cartoonist, publisher and Aviation School trainer, ex- moderator on Medico.in, banker, student councilor ,travelogue writer … among other things! One fine morning, she decided that she had enough of killing herself by Degrees and went back to her first love -- writing. It's more enjoyable! She already has 48 published academic and 14 fiction- in- different- genre books under her belt.

When she is not designing websites or making Graphic design illustrations for clients , she is browsing through old bookshops hunting for treasures, of which she has an enviable collection – including R.L. Stevenson, O.Henry, Dornford Yates, Maurice Walsh, C.N.Williamson, Sapper, Bartimeus and the crown of her collection- Dickens "The Old Curiosity Shop," and so on… Just call her "Renaissance Woman" - collecting herbal remedies, acting like Universal Helping Hand/Agony Aunt, or escaping to her dear mountains for a bit of exploring, collecting herbs and plants, and trekking.

Check out some of the other Health Learning Series books at Amazon.com

Health Learning Series on Amazon

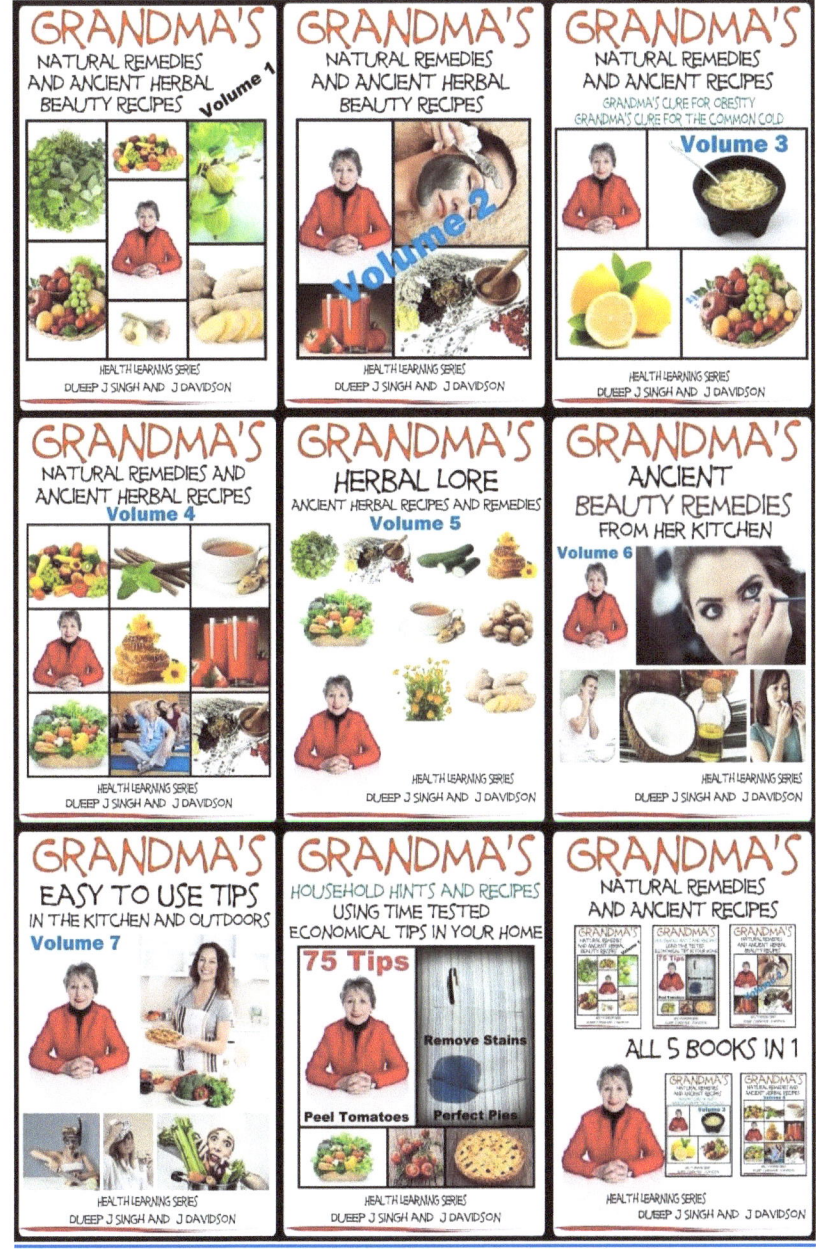

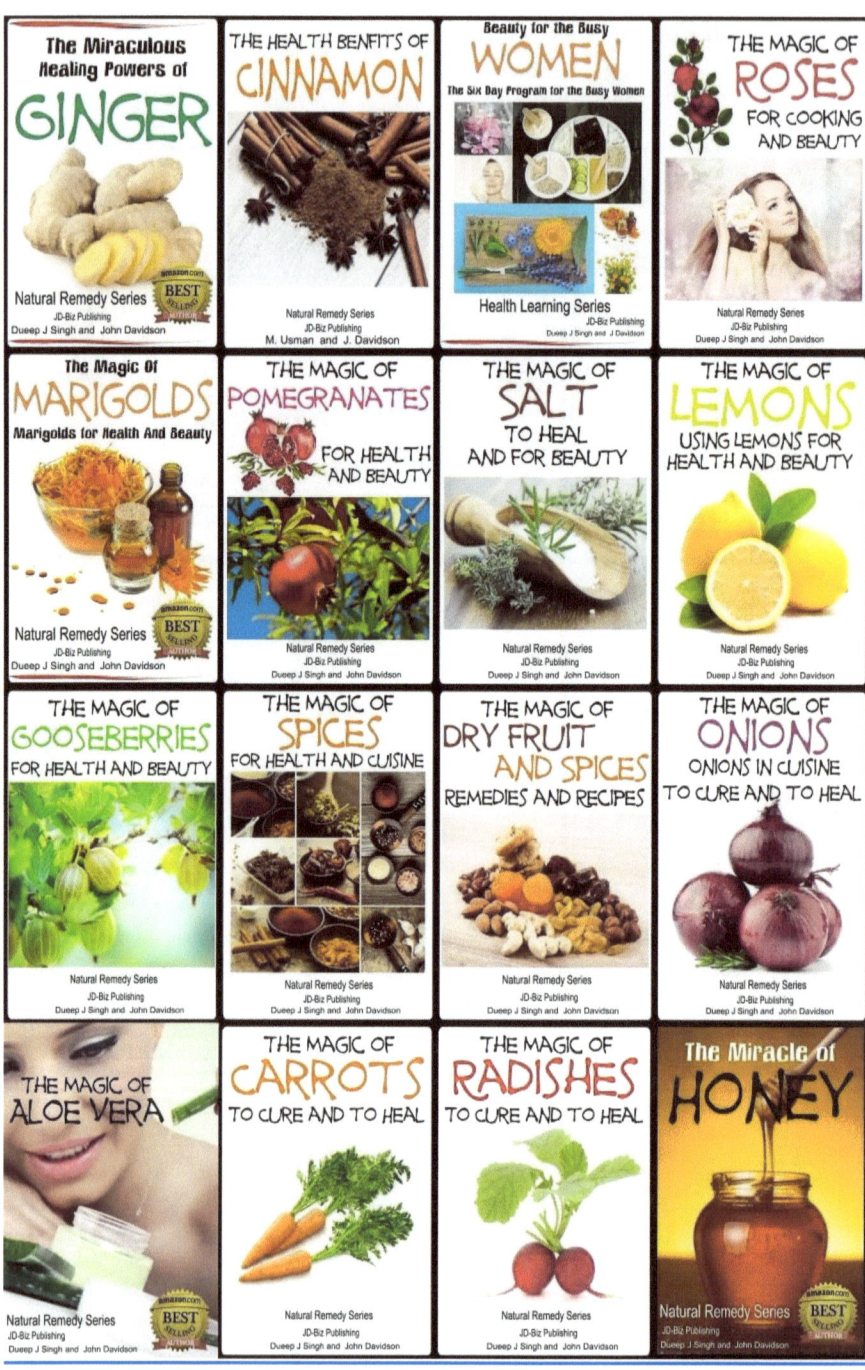

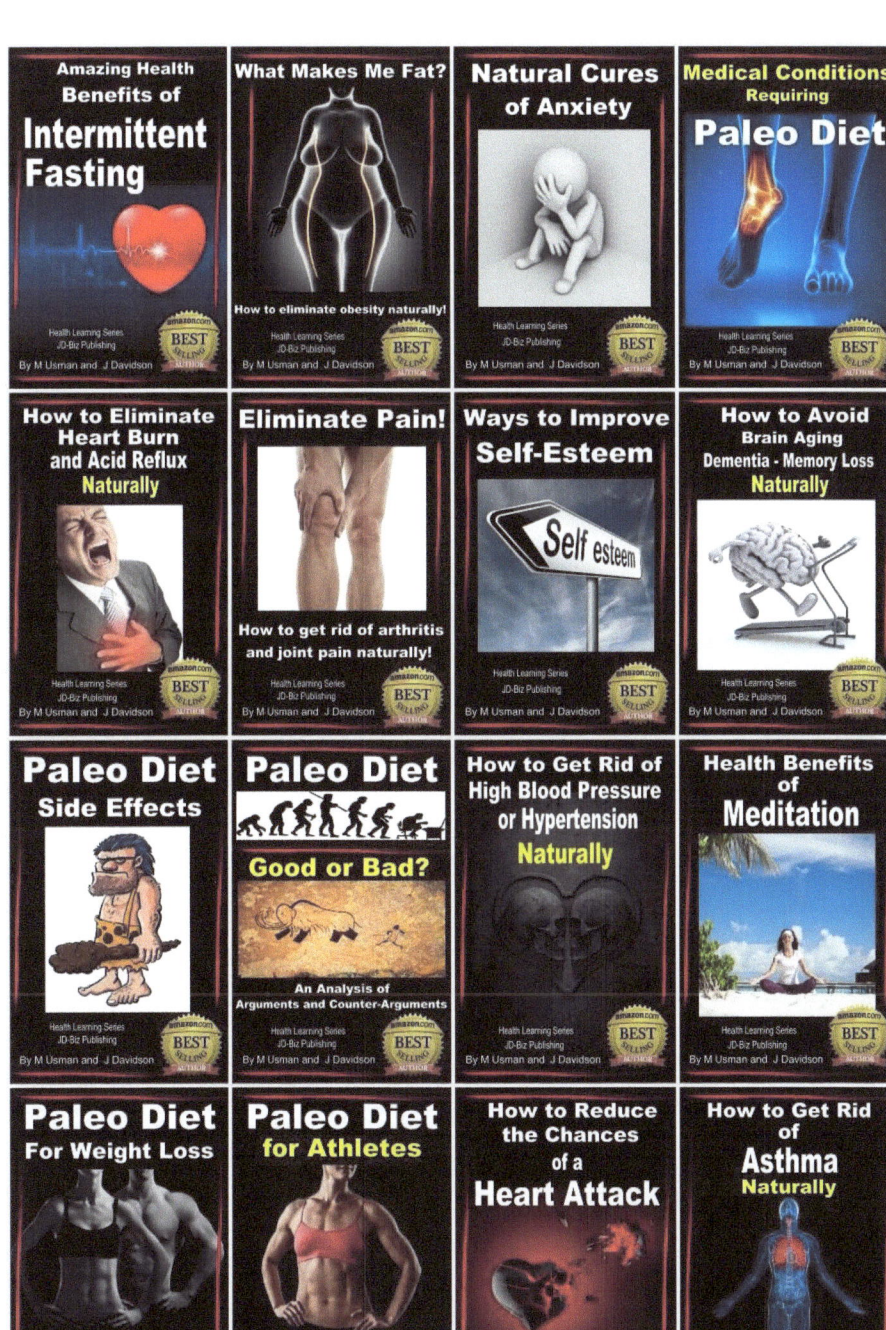

Amazing Animal Books Series

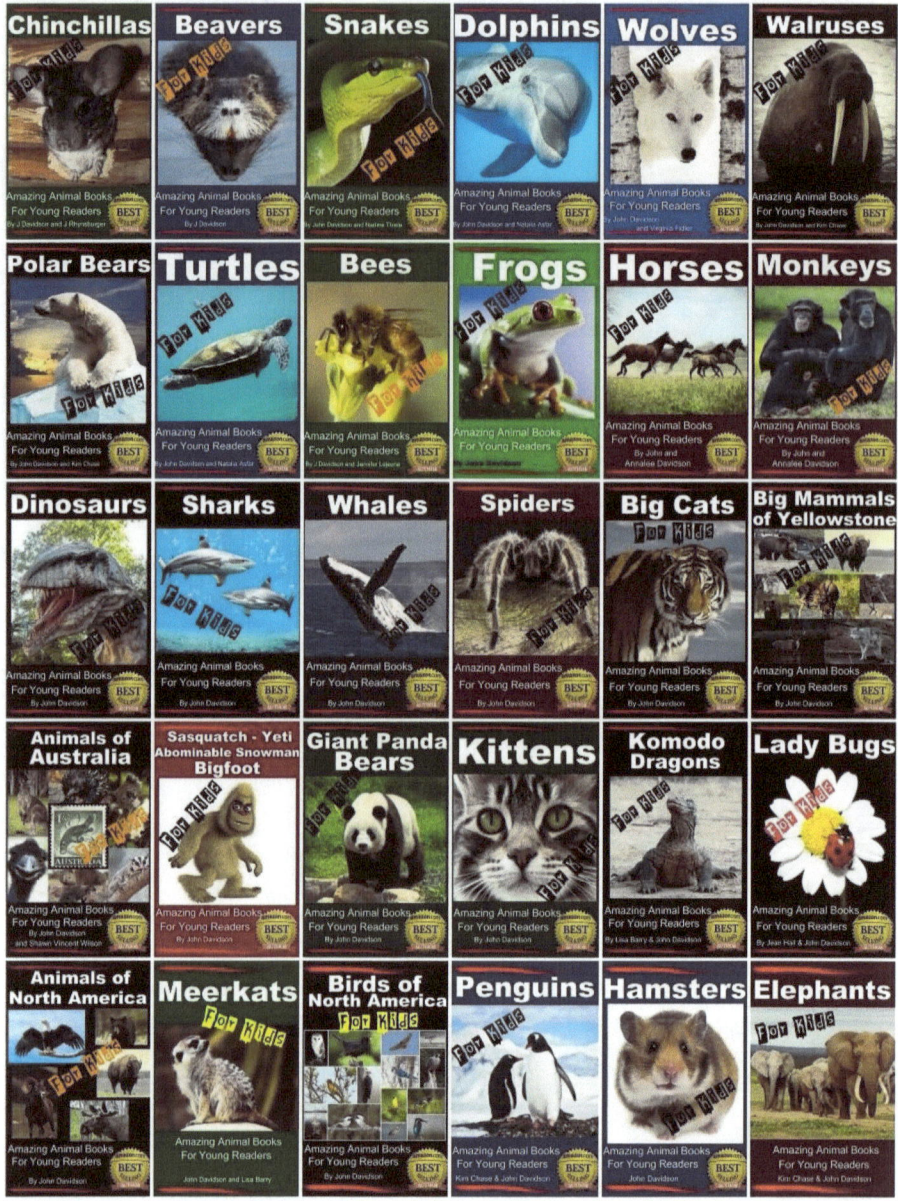

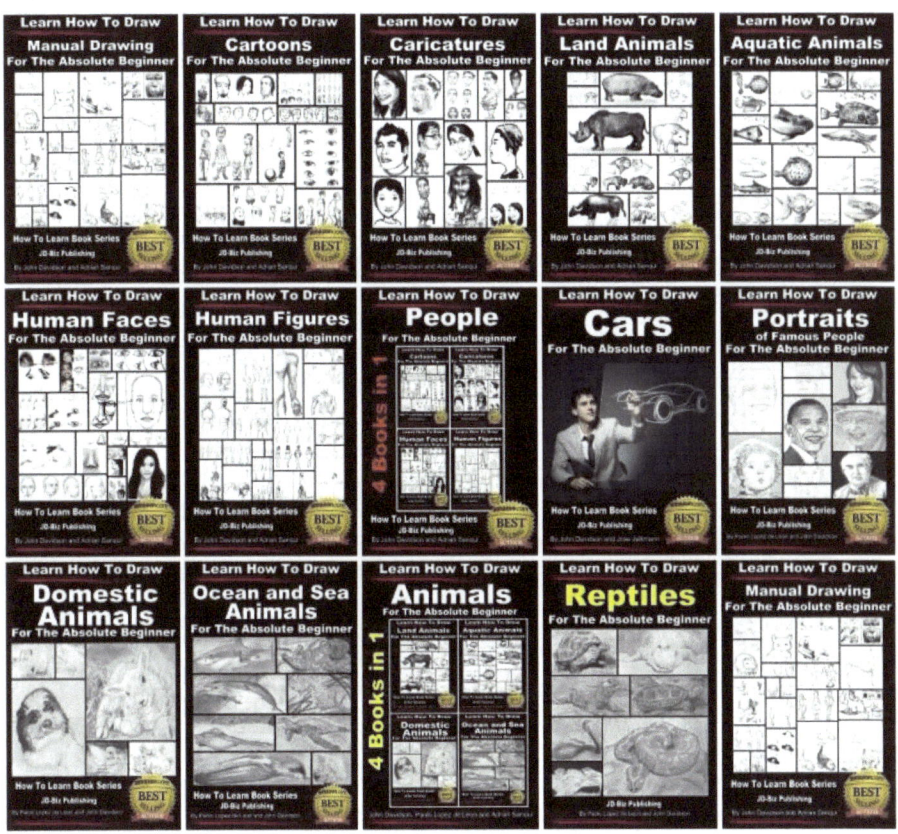

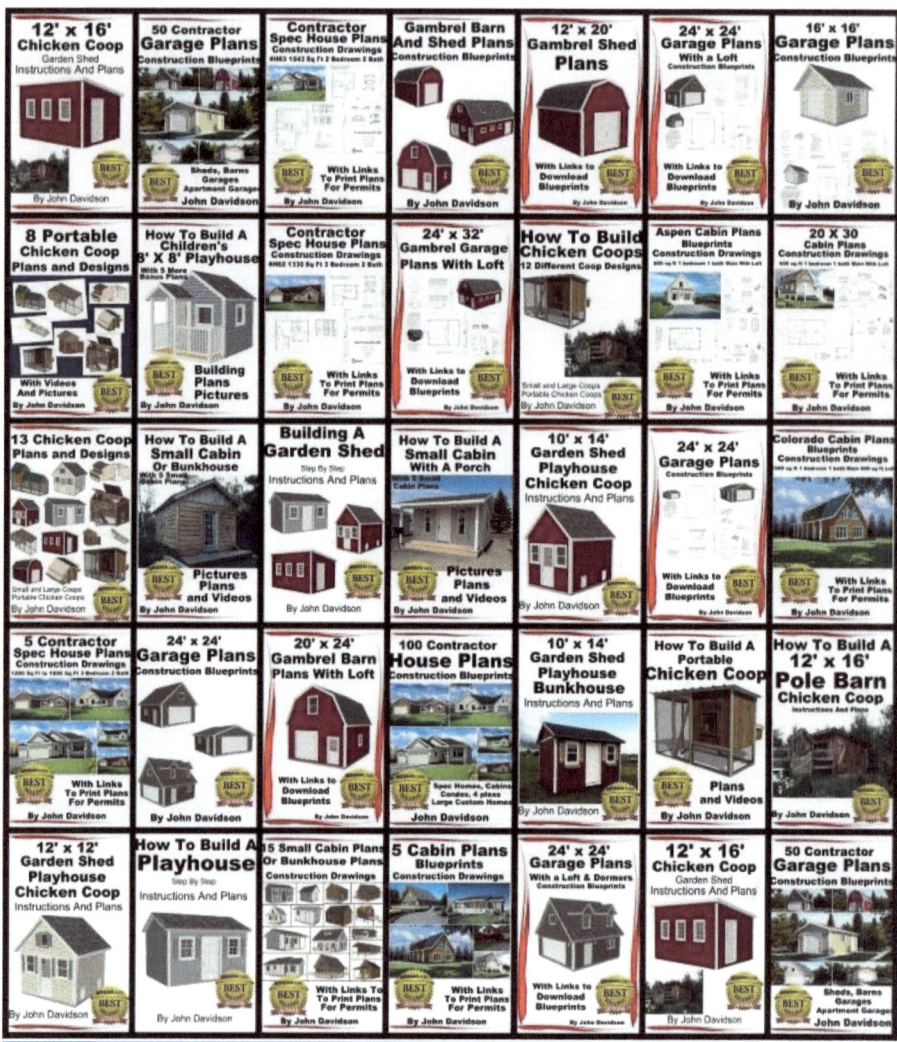

Our books are available at

1. Amazon.com

2. Barnes and Noble

3. Itunes

4. Kobo

5. Smashwords

6. Google Play Books

Download Free Books!

http://MendonCottageBooks.com

Publisher

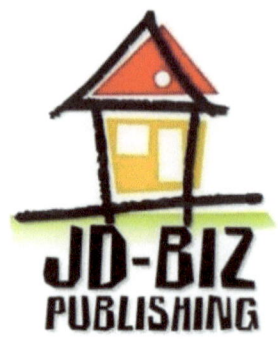

JD-Biz Corp

P O Box 374

Mendon, Utah 84325

http://www.jd-biz.com/

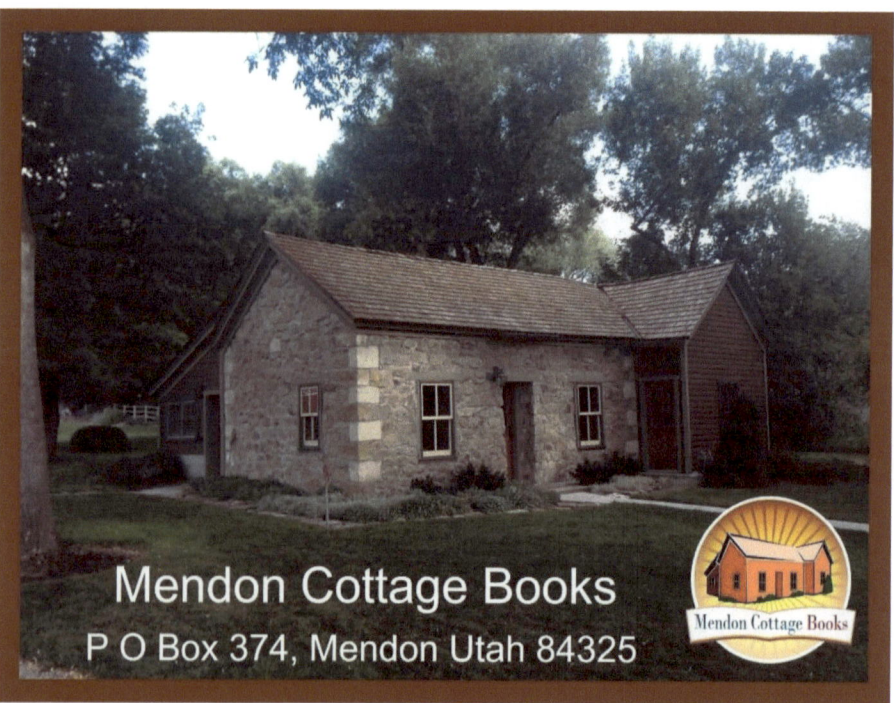